I0844008

NATURAL REMEDIES FOR DIGESTIVE HEALTH

Healthy Choices For Gut Health and Improved Digestion

RUTH PETERS

Copyright © 2023 by Ruth Peters

All rights reserved.

TABLE OF CONTENT

INTRODUCTION

In a world filled with hustle and bustle, where time races forward and stress pulls you in every direction, there's one silent hero often overlooked – your digestive system. Picture this: a bustling marketplace of nutrients, enzymes, and bacteria, working harmoniously to process your meals, converting them into fuel for your journey through life.

But what happens when this marketplace becomes a chaotic scene? When the gates of your digestive system are thrown open to unhealthy choices, irregular eating habits, and the weight of modern pressures? It's then that your internal world mirrors the chaos of the external, leaving you feeling sluggish, uncomfortable, and out of sync.

Imagine standing at the crossroads of this bustling market, armed not with pharmaceuticals or quick fixes, but with the wisdom of nature itself. Here begins our exploration – "Natural Remedies for Digestive Health." In this book, we'll embark on a journey that unveils the secret treasures nature offers to bring harmony back to your body.

From the enchanting gardens of herbal remedies to the kitchens filled with nourishing foods, and the tranquil corners where ancient practices meet modern wisdom. You'll discover the power of peppermint leaves to soothe, ginger roots to invigorate, and chamomile flowers to calm. We'll navigate the labyrinth of dietary choices, learning how fibers dance through your systems and how the right bacteria can orchestrate a symphony of wellness.

We'll delve into the art of mindful eating, where every bite becomes a moment of meditation, and we'll unravel the threads connecting gut and stress, unveiling the undeniable truth: a calm mind nurtures a peaceful belly, we'll gather homemade remedies, blending ancient traditions with contemporary lifestyles.

So, dear reader, open these pages with curiosity and hope, let's venture forth together into the realm of natural remedies for digestive health, where each turn of the page brings you closer to reclaiming the vitality and equilibrium that is rightfully yours

CHAPTER 1

UNDERSTANDING DIGESTIVE SYSTEM

The digestive system is like a well-coordinated factory that processes the food we eat, breaking it down into nutrients our body can use for energy, growth, and repair. It's a complex system involving various organs and processes working together seamlessly.

Here's how it works:

Mouth

The digestive process begins in the mouth. As you chew, your salivary glands release enzymes that start breaking down starches. The food forms a ball called a **bolus**, which you then swallow.

Esophagus

The bolus moves down the esophagus, a muscular tube, via a series of coordinated contractions called **peristalsis**.

Stomach

The bolus enters the stomach, where gastric juices containing hydrochloric acid and enzymes help break down proteins. The stomach's churning motion further mixes the food and juices, forming a semi-liquid substance called **chyme**.

Small Intestine

The chyme enters the small intestine, where most of the digestion and absorption occur. Here, bile from the liver and enzymes from the pancreas help break down fats, proteins, and carbohydrates into smaller molecules that can be absorbed into the bloodstream.

Large Intestine

The remaining undigested food and waste move into the large intestine. Water and electrolytes are absorbed here, and beneficial bacteria help further break down certain substances. The result is the formation of feces.

Rectum and Anus

Feces are stored in the rectum until they are eliminated through the anus during a bowel movement.

Throughout this process, various hormones, nerves, and reflexes work together to regulate digestion and ensure that nutrients are properly absorbed while waste products are eliminated. This intricate system not only fuels our bodies but also plays a crucial role in maintaining overall health.

Maintaining a balanced diet, staying hydrated, and adopting healthy eating habits can contribute to a smoothly functioning digestive system and a healthier life overall.

COMMON DIGESTIVE ISSUES

Our digestive system, though remarkable, isn't immune to challenges. Various factors like diet, lifestyle, genetics, and stress can lead to a range of digestive issues. Understanding these issues can empower you to take preventive measures and seek timely medical advice when needed.

Acid Reflux/GERD

Acid reflux, also known as gastroesophageal reflux disease (GERD), is a common digestive disorder where stomach acid flows back into the esophagus, causing discomfort and irritation. This occurs due to a weakened lower esophageal sphincter (LES), a muscular ring that usually prevents acid from entering the esophagus. Symptoms often include heartburn, a burning sensation in the chest, regurgitation of sour-tasting fluids, and sometimes, a persistent cough.

GERD can result from various factors including diet choices, obesity, smoking, and pregnancy. Certain foods, like spicy or acidic ones, caffeine, and fatty meals, can trigger symptoms. If left untreated, GERD can lead to complications such as esophagitis (inflammation of the esophagus), ulcers, and even an increased risk of esophageal cancer.

Managing GERD involves lifestyle changes like avoiding trigger foods, eating smaller meals, not lying down after eating, and maintaining a healthy weight.

Irritable Bowel Syndrome (IBS)

Irritable bowel syndrome (IBS) is a common gastrointestinal disorder that affects the large intestine. It's characterized by a combination of symptoms, including abdominal pain, bloating, gas, diarrhea, and constipation. The exact cause of IBS is not fully understood, but factors like sensitive nerves in the gut, muscle contractions, and changes in gut bacteria might play a role.

IBS is often triggered or exacerbated by certain foods, stress, hormonal changes, or infections. Symptoms can vary from person to person and may come and go over time. While IBS can be uncomfortable and disruptive, it doesn't cause permanent damage to the intestines or increase the risk of more serious conditions like inflammatory bowel disease or cancer.

Managing IBS involves a personalized approach. Dietary modifications, such as avoiding trigger foods (like certain types of carbohydrates) and increasing fiber intake, can help regulate bowel movements. Stress reduction techniques, regular exercise, and maintaining a consistent eating schedule can also contribute to symptom relief. In some cases, doctors might recommend medications to alleviate specific symptoms.

Inflammatory Bowel Disease (IBD)

Inflammatory bowel disease (IBD) is a group of chronic disorders that cause inflammation in the digestive tract. The two main types of IBD are Crohn's disease and ulcerative colitis. These conditions involve the immune system mistakenly attacking the lining of the intestines, leading to inflammation, ulcers, and various gastrointestinal symptoms.

Crohn's disease can affect any part of the digestive tract and may result in abdominal pain, diarrhea, weight loss, and fatigue. Ulcerative colitis primarily affects the colon and rectum, causing symptoms like bloody diarrhea, abdominal pain, and urgency to have bowel movements.

The exact cause of IBD is complex and involves genetic, environmental, and immune system factors. While there's no cure, treatments aim to manage symptoms and reduce inflammation. Medications, lifestyle changes, and in some cases, surgery, may be necessary. IBD can have significant impacts on daily life, but with proper medical care and support, individuals can lead fulfilling lives.

Celiac Disease

Celiac disease is an autoimmune disorder triggered by consuming gluten, a protein found in wheat, barley, and rye. When someone with celiac disease eats gluten, their immune system responds by damaging the lining of the small intestine. This impairs nutrient absorption and can lead to a range of symptoms.

Symptoms vary widely and may include digestive issues like diarrhea, bloating, and abdominal pain, as well as non-digestive symptoms such as fatigue, joint pain, skin rashes, and mood disturbances. Over time, untreated celiac disease can lead to malnutrition and related health problems.

The only effective treatment for celiac disease is adopting a strict gluten-free diet. This means avoiding all foods and products containing wheat, barley, and rye derivatives. Incorporating naturally gluten-free grains like rice, corn, and quinoa is important for maintaining a balanced diet.

Constipation

Constipation refers to infrequent or difficult bowel movements, often accompanied by hard, dry stools. It's a common digestive issue caused by various factors, including inadequate fiber intake, insufficient hydration, lack of physical activity, and certain medications. Stress and certain medical conditions can also contribute.

Symptoms of constipation may include straining during bowel movements, a feeling of incomplete evacuation, abdominal discomfort, and reduced bowel frequency. While occasional constipation is normal, chronic constipation can lead to discomfort and impact daily life.

Preventing constipation involves maintaining a balanced diet rich in fiber from fruits, vegetables, whole grains, and legumes. Staying well-hydrated and engaging in regular physical activity can also help regulate bowel movements. In some cases, over-the-counter fiber supplements might be recommended.

Diarrhea

Diarrhea is a common digestive issue characterized by loose, watery stools occurring more frequently than usual. It can result from infections (bacterial, viral, or parasitic), food intolerances, medications, and underlying medical conditions. Diarrhea occurs when the intestines don't absorb sufficient water or when excessive fluid is secreted into the intestines.

Symptoms of diarrhea may include frequent bowel movements, urgency to use the restroom, abdominal cramps, and dehydration due to fluid loss. While usually short-lived and not serious, persistent or severe diarrhea can lead to complications like dehydration and nutrient deficiencies.

Gallstones

Gallstones are small, solid particles that form in the gallbladder, a small organ located beneath the liver. They develop when substances in the bile, such as cholesterol and bilirubin, become imbalanced and crystallize. Gallstones can range in size from tiny grains to larger masses.

While many people with gallstones may not experience any symptoms, when a stone blocks the flow of bile from the gallbladder, it can lead to intense pain, known as a gallbladder attack. This pain often occurs in the upper right abdomen and can radiate to the back or right shoulder. Nausea, vomiting, and discomfort after fatty meals are common symptoms.

Gallstones are associated with factors like obesity, a high-fat diet, rapid weight loss, pregnancy, and genetics.

Lactose Intolerance

Lactose intolerance is a digestive disorder where the body can't fully digest lactose, a sugar found in milk and dairy products. This occurs due to insufficient levels of lactase, an enzyme needed to break down lactose in the small intestine. As a result, undigested lactose can lead to symptoms like bloating, gas, diarrhea, and abdominal discomfort.

Symptoms usually occur within a few hours of consuming lactose-containing foods. They can vary in severity depending on the amount of lactose consumed and an individual's tolerance level. Lactose intolerance is different from a milk allergy, which involves the immune system reacting to milk proteins.

Managing lactose intolerance involves dietary adjustments. Many people with lactose intolerance can tolerate small amounts of lactose without symptoms. Lactase supplements, available over-the-counter, can help digest lactose when taken before consuming dairy. Lactose-free and dairy-free alternatives are also widely available.

Diverticulitis

Diverticulitis is a condition where small pouches (diverticula) that can form in the walls of the colon become inflamed or infected. It's often linked to a condition called diverticulosis, where these pouches develop over time due to weak spots in the colon wall. Diverticulitis can cause abdominal pain, usually on the left side, along with fever, nausea, vomiting, and changes in bowel habits.

While the exact cause isn't fully understood, a diet low in fiber is believed to contribute to the development of diverticulosis and the risk of diverticulitis. Fiber helps maintain regular bowel movements and prevent inflammation and infection of the pouches.

Peptic Ulcers

Peptic ulcers are open sores that develop on the inner lining of the stomach, small intestine, or esophagus. These ulcers can be painful and cause discomfort. They typically form due to an imbalance between stomach acids and protective factors in the digestive tract.

Common causes include infection with the bacterium Helicobacter pylori, prolonged use of nonsteroidal anti-inflammatory drugs (NSAIDs), excessive stomach acid production, and lifestyle factors like smoking and excessive alcohol consumption. Symptoms can include burning stomach pain, bloating, heartburn, and nausea.

Treatment includes medications to reduce stomach acid production, antibiotics if H. pylori infection is present, and lifestyle modifications such as quitting smoking and avoiding triggers like NSAIDs.

Peptic ulcers can lead to serious complications if left untreated, such as bleeding or perforation of the stomach or intestine. With proper treatment and lifestyle adjustments, most peptic ulcers can heal, and recurrence can be minimized.

BENEFITS OF NATURAL REMEDIES

Natural remedies offer a range of benefits for maintaining and improving overall health. Here's an overview of their advantages:

Gentle Approach: Natural remedies often work in harmony with the body's natural processes, supporting healing without causing harsh side effects or disruptions.

Minimal Side Effects: Compared to pharmaceutical medications, natural remedies generally have fewer and milder side effects, making them a safer option for many individuals.

Holistic Healing: Natural remedies often consider the whole person — physical, mental, and emotional aspects. This holistic approach can contribute to overall well-being.

Nourishing Nutrients: Many natural remedies, like herbal teas, are rich in vitamins, minerals, and antioxidants that provide essential nutrients for the body.

Supporting the Body's Defense: Some natural remedies, such as certain herbs, can help boost the immune system and enhance the body's ability to fight off illnesses.

Digestive Harmony: Natural remedies like ginger, peppermint, and fennel can promote healthy digestion, reducing issues like bloating, indigestion, and gas.

Reduced Chemical Exposure: Natural remedies often involve using whole, unprocessed ingredients, reducing exposure to artificial chemicals and additives.

Personalized Approach: Natural remedies can be tailored to individual needs, allowing for a more personalized and effective treatment plan.

Long-Term Benefits: Natural remedies often aim to address the root cause of issues rather than just masking symptoms, leading to long-term improvements.

Mind-Body Connection: Many natural remedies incorporate practices like meditation, yoga, and relaxation techniques that can positively impact both mental and physical health.

Sustainability: Using natural remedies often aligns with environmentally friendly practices, promoting sustainability and reducing the ecological footprint.

Cultural Wisdom: Natural remedies draw from centuries of traditional knowledge passed down through generations, incorporating cultural wisdom and practices.

Affordability: Natural remedies can be more cost-effective than pharmaceutical medications, making health management more accessible.

Empowerment: Learning about and using natural remedies empowers individuals to take an active role in their health and well-being.

Complementary Options: Natural remedies can complement conventional medical treatments, providing additional support and improving overall outcomes.

Take note, while natural remedies can offer numerous benefits, it's important to approach them with knowledge and caution. Consulting with healthcare professionals before incorporating new remedies, especially if you have existing health conditions or are on medications, is a wise practice. Additionally, natural remedies might not be suitable for all situations, so a balanced approach that considers various treatment options is recommended.

CHAPTER 2

HERBAL REMEDIES

In this chapter, we will explore different versatile herbs, that aids digestive health.

PEPPERMINT

Peppermint (Mentha x piperita) is a versatile herb known for its refreshing aroma and a wide array of medicinal properties. When it comes to digestive health, peppermint stands as a stalwart ally, offering relief from various discomforts and promoting overall gastrointestinal wellness.

How Peppermint Works

Peppermint owes its digestive benefits to its active compound, menthol. Menthol has a soothing effect on the muscles of the gastrointestinal tract, helping to relax spasms and reduce cramping. It also helps to increase the flow of bile, aiding in the digestion of fats. This dual action makes peppermint particularly effective in managing conditions like irritable bowel syndrome (IBS) where spasms and discomfort are common.

Benefits for Digestive Health:

Relief from Indigestion: Peppermint can provide relief from indigestion by relaxing the muscles of the stomach and promoting the flow of bile. This can ease symptoms like bloating, gas, and discomfort after meals.

Alleviation of IBS Symptoms: Peppermint oil capsules have been extensively studied for their ability to alleviate symptoms of irritable bowel syndrome, including abdominal pain, bloating, and altered bowel habits.

Soothing Effect on Heartburn: The cooling sensation of menthol can help soothe the burning sensation of heartburn by calming the lower esophageal sphincter.

Reduction of Nausea: Peppermint's aroma and compounds can have a calming effect on the stomach, helping to reduce feelings of nausea and vomiting.

Ways to Incorporate Peppermint:

Peppermint Tea: A soothing cup of peppermint tea can ease digestion after a meal and provide relaxation.

Peppermint Oil: Peppermint oil capsules, when taken as directed, can be effective in managing IBS symptoms.

Aromatherapy: Inhaling the aroma of peppermint essential oil can have a calming effect on the stomach and reduce feelings of nausea.

Precautions

While peppermint is generally safe for most people, it's essential to exercise caution if you have acid reflux or gastroesophageal reflux disease (GERD). In some cases, peppermint can relax the lower esophageal sphincter, potentially worsening symptoms. Additionally, if you're considering peppermint oil capsules, consult a healthcare professional, especially if you have underlying health conditions or are taking medications.

Peppermint offers a delightful and effective natural remedy for a range of digestive discomforts. Its soothing properties can make a noticeable difference in your digestive well-being. However, as with any herbal remedy, it's wise to approach its use with awareness and consideration of your individual health needs.

GINGER

Ginger (Zingiber officinale) is not just a kitchen spice; it's a powerful herbal remedy revered for its multitude of health benefits, especially in promoting digestive wellness. Known for centuries for its medicinal properties, ginger continues to captivate with its remarkable ability to soothe various digestive discomforts.

How Ginger Supports Digestion:

Ginger owes its digestive prowess to its bioactive compounds, notably gingerol. These compounds are responsible for ginger's anti-inflammatory, antioxidant, and antiemetic (anti-nausea) effects. By stimulating the digestive system and soothing inflammation, ginger can be

a valuable asset in maintaining gut
health.

Benefits for Digestive Health:

Alleviation of Nausea and Vomiting:
Ginger's antiemetic properties are
well-documented, making it a trusted
natural remedy for motion sickness,
morning sickness during pregnancy,
and chemotherapy-induced nausea.

Relief from Indigestion: Ginger's
ability to increase digestive juices and
neutralize stomach acids can ease
symptoms of indigestion, such as
bloating, discomfort, and heartburn.

**Soothing for Irritable Bowel
Syndrome (IBS):** Ginger's anti-
inflammatory effects can help reduce
inflammation in the gut, offering relief

to those with irritable bowel syndrome.

Motion Sickness: Whether by land, air, or sea, ginger's ability to calm the stomach makes it a reliable remedy for motion sickness.

Ways to Incorporate Ginger:

Ginger Tea: A warm cup of ginger tea can be soothing for digestion and offer relief from nausea. Simply steep fresh ginger slices in hot water.

Ginger Chews or Candies: These portable options can be a convenient way to keep ginger on hand for whenever nausea strikes.

Cooking with Ginger: Adding fresh ginger to your meals, whether in stir-fries, soups, or marinades, can infuse your dishes with its flavor and health benefits.

Ginger Supplements: Ginger supplements in the form of capsules or extracts are also available, but it's advisable to consult a healthcare professional before adding supplements to your routine.

Precautions

While ginger is considered safe for most people, consuming excessive amounts might lead to digestive discomfort or heartburn. If you're considering using ginger for medicinal purposes, especially if you're pregnant, have underlying health conditions, or take medications, it's wise to consult a healthcare professional. Also, be mindful of potential interactions if you're on blood-thinning medications.

Ginger's remarkable versatility extends far beyond its culinary appeal. As a natural digestive aid, it has rightfully earned its place in the realm of herbal remedies, offering relief and comfort to those seeking gentle, effective solutions for various digestive concerns.

CHAMOMILE

Chamomile (Matricaria chamomilla) is more than just a soothing bedtime tea; it's a botanical wonder revered for its calming properties and extensive health benefits. In the realm of digestive health, chamomile shines as a gentle yet potent remedy, offering relief from a range of discomforts and promoting overall well-being.

How Chamomile Nurtures Digestion:

Chamomile's magic lies in its bioactive compounds, including apigenin and chamazulene. These compounds possess anti-inflammatory, antispasmodic, and relaxant properties that work harmoniously to ease digestive distress and promote relaxation within the gastrointestinal tract.

Benefits for Digestive Health:

Calm for Upset Stomach:
Chamomile's natural antispasmodic

properties can provide relief from stomach cramps, bloating, and gas, calming the tumultuous tides of an upset stomach.

Aid for Indigestion: Chamomile's gentle bitterness stimulates digestive juices, helping to alleviate indigestion symptoms like discomfort and fullness.

Relief from Nausea: Sipping chamomile tea can have a soothing effect on the stomach, making it a go-to option for quelling feelings of nausea.

Anti-Inflammatory Support: The anti-inflammatory compounds in chamomile can help reduce inflammation in the digestive tract, offering relief for conditions like irritable bowel syndrome (IBS).

Ways to Embrace Chamomile:

Chamomile Tea: The classic option, chamomile tea is easy to prepare and offers warmth and comfort for digestion. Steep dried chamomile flowers in hot water for a few minutes.

Chamomile Infusions: Beyond tea, you can infuse chamomile in water, creating a mild tonic to sip throughout the day.

Chamomile Essential Oil: Aromatherapy with chamomile essential oil can have a relaxing effect on both the mind and the digestive system.

Chamomile Supplements: Capsules or tinctures containing chamomile extracts are available, but consulting a healthcare professional before using supplements is advised.

Precautions:

Chamomile is generally safe for most people, but if you have allergies to plants in the Asteraceae family (ragweed, marigolds, daisies), exercise caution. Also, if you're pregnant, nursing, or taking medications, consult a healthcare professional before using chamomile in medicinal amounts.

Chamomile's gentle nature and versatile applications make it an enchanting addition to the world of herbal remedies. From calming an uneasy stomach to offering a soothing ritual for relaxation, chamomile's embrace is gentle yet transformative for digestive well-being.

ALOE VERA

Aloe vera (Aloe barbadensis miller) isn't just a soothing balm for skin; it's also a revered herbal remedy with a longstanding history of aiding digestive health. Known for its soothing and healing properties, aloe vera extends its beneficial touch to the intricate realm of the digestive system, offering relief and support for various concerns.

How Aloe Vera Nurtures Digestion:

Aloe vera's gel contains bioactive compounds, including polysaccharides and anthraquinones, that contribute to its anti-inflammatory, soothing, and protective effects. These compounds work synergistically to promote digestive wellness and provide comfort to an array of digestive discomforts.

Benefits for Digestive Health:

Gentle Relief for Heartburn: Aloe vera's cooling properties can help alleviate the burning sensation of heartburn by soothing the esophagus.

Support for Irritable Bowel Syndrome (IBS): Aloe vera's anti-inflammatory effects may offer relief to those with IBS, helping to calm gut inflammation and discomfort.

Promotion of Regularity: Aloe vera's gentle laxative effect can aid in promoting regular bowel movements, making it helpful for mild cases of constipation.

Soothing for Gastric Ulcers: Aloe vera's protective properties may contribute to the healing of gastric ulcers by reducing inflammation and promoting tissue repair.

Ways to Experience Aloe Vera:

Aloe Vera Juice: Consuming aloe vera juice (pure and without additives) can provide a range of digestive benefits. However, moderation is key, as excessive consumption might lead to laxative effects.

Aloe Vera Gel: Aloe vera gel can be consumed directly or added to smoothies and beverages. Be cautious about the quantity to avoid laxative effects.

Aloe Vera Supplements: Aloe vera supplements, available in various forms, provide the benefits of aloe vera without the need for consuming large quantities. Consult a healthcare professional before using supplements.

Precautions

While aloe vera offers remarkable benefits, it's important to exercise caution, as excessive consumption can lead to adverse effects like diarrhea and electrolyte imbalances. If you're pregnant, nursing, have underlying health conditions, or are taking medications, consult a healthcare professional before using aloe vera for medicinal purposes.

Aloe vera's versatile healing touch extends from the outside in, nurturing digestive health and offering relief from various discomforts. With its array of soothing and protective properties, aloe vera stands as a cherished companion in the journey toward digestive balance.

FENNEL

Fennel (Foeniculum vulgare) is more than just a flavorful addition to recipes; it's a cherished herb that has been revered for centuries for its culinary and medicinal properties. When it comes to digestive health, fennel stands as a gentle yet effective remedy, offering relief from a variety of discomforts and promoting digestive harmony.

How Fennel Supports Digestion:

Fennel owes its digestive benefits to its unique blend of compounds, including anethole and fenchone. These compounds possess antispasmodic, carminative, and anti-inflammatory properties, which work in tandem to soothe the digestive system and alleviate discomfort.

Benefits for Digestive Health:

Aid for Bloating and Gas: Fennel's natural carminative properties can help reduce bloating, gas, and abdominal discomfort by relaxing the muscles of the gastrointestinal tract.

Relief from Indigestion: Fennel seeds can stimulate the production of digestive juices, aiding in the digestion of fats and alleviating symptoms of indigestion.

Calming Effect for IBS: Fennel's antispasmodic effects can provide relief from spasms and discomfort associated with irritable bowel syndrome (IBS).

Support for Acid Reflux: Chewing fennel seeds after meals can help neutralize excess stomach acid, offering relief from acid reflux.

Ways to Enjoy Fennel

Fennel Tea: A soothing cup of fennel tea can provide comfort after meals and ease digestive discomfort. Simply steep crushed fennel seeds in hot water.

Fennel Seeds: Chewing on a teaspoon of fennel seeds after meals can aid digestion and offer relief from bloating and gas.

Cooking with Fennel: Incorporate fresh fennel bulbs, seeds, or fennel leaves into your culinary creations to infuse dishes with its aromatic flavor.

Fennel Oil: Fennel essential oil can be used in aromatherapy or diluted for massage to ease digestive discomfort.

Precautions

Fennel is generally safe for most people, but individuals with allergies to celery, carrot, or mugwort might experience cross-reactivity. If you're pregnant, nursing, taking medications, or have a history of seizures or estrogen-sensitive conditions, consult a healthcare professional before using fennel supplements or essential oil.

Fennel's gentle and aromatic touch adds not only flavor to cuisine but also a sense of comfort to the digestive journey. As a trusted ally in promoting digestion and alleviating discomfort, fennel embodies the harmony between the culinary and the medicinal.

LICORICE ROOT

Licorice root (Glycyrrhiza glabra) is more than just a sweet treat; it's a powerful herbal remedy with a rich history in traditional medicine. Renowned for its natural sweetness and a host of medicinal compounds, licorice root plays a vital role in promoting digestive health, offering relief from various discomforts, and nurturing overall well-being.

How Licorice Root Nurtures Digestion

Licorice root contains compounds like glycyrrhizin and flavonoids, which contribute to its anti-inflammatory, soothing, and protective effects. These compounds work in synergy to support digestive health and provide comfort for a range of digestive issues.

Benefits for Digestive Health:

Gentle Relief for Acid Reflux: Licorice root's soothing properties can help alleviate the discomfort of acid reflux by forming a protective coating in the esophagus.

Calming Effect for Irritable Bowel Syndrome (IBS): Licorice root's anti-inflammatory and antispasmodic effects can provide relief from spasms and discomfort associated with IBS.

Protection for Gastric Ulcers: Licorice root's compounds may help stimulate the production of mucus in the stomach, offering a protective barrier for gastric ulcers.

Alleviation of Bloating and Gas: Licorice root's natural anti-inflammatory properties can help reduce bloating, gas, and abdominal discomfort.

Ways to Experience Licorice Root:

Licorice Tea: A cup of licorice tea can be soothing for digestion and offer relief from discomfort. Opt for deglycyrrhizinated licorice (DGL) tea to avoid potential side effects of glycyrrhizin.

DGL Supplements: Deglycyrrhizinated licorice supplements are available in tablet or chewable form and can provide the benefits of licorice root without the potential for excessive glycyrrhizin intake.

Licorice Extract: Licorice root extract, when used cautiously and under the guidance of a healthcare professional, can provide concentrated benefits.

Precautions

While licorice root offers numerous benefits, it's important to exercise caution. The compound glycyrrhizin in licorice root can lead to potential side effects like high blood pressure and potassium imbalances, especially with excessive consumption. Pregnant and breastfeeding individuals, those with high blood pressure, and those taking medications should consult a healthcare professional before using licorice root in medicinal amounts.

Licorice root's sweet embrace extends beyond its flavor, offering a soothing touch to digestive concerns. With its diverse applications and array of beneficial compounds, licorice root stands as a potent ally in nurturing digestive harmony and promoting overall well-being.

CLOVES

Cloves (Syzygium aromaticum) are more than just a fragrant spice; they are a prized herbal remedy known for their potent aroma and rich array of medicinal properties. In the realm of digestive health, cloves shine as a versatile ally, offering relief from discomforts and promoting overall well-being.

How Cloves Work Their Magic

Cloves owe their digestive benefits to their bioactive compounds, including eugenol. Eugenol is responsible for cloves' antimicrobial, anti-inflammatory, and analgesic properties, making them a dynamic choice for addressing various digestive concerns.

Benefits for Digestive Health

Soothing for Indigestion: Cloves' aromatic properties can stimulate the production of digestive enzymes, helping to alleviate symptoms of indigestion like bloating and discomfort.

Relief from Gas and Bloating: Cloves' carminative properties can help reduce gas and bloating by promoting the expulsion of excess air from the digestive tract.

Aid for Nausea and Vomiting: Cloves' aromatic fragrance can have a calming effect on the stomach, providing relief from nausea and vomiting.

Antimicrobial Support: Cloves' natural antimicrobial properties can help combat harmful microorganisms in the digestive tract, promoting a healthy gut environment.

Ways to Incorporate Cloves

Cloves in Cooking: Adding whole cloves to your culinary creations, such as stews, rice dishes, and desserts, can infuse your meals with their aromatic flavor.

Cloves Tea: Cloves tea, made by steeping whole or ground cloves in hot water, can offer a soothing beverage for digestion.

Cloves Oil: Cloves essential oil, when diluted appropriately, can be used for aromatherapy or massage to ease digestive discomfort.

Precautions

While cloves offer remarkable benefits, their strong flavor and potency should be used in moderation. If you're pregnant, nursing, have underlying health conditions, or take medications, consult a healthcare professional before using cloves in medicinal amounts or in the form of essential oil.

Cloves' aromatic allure goes beyond the kitchen, offering a comforting touch to digestive woes. With their unique blend of beneficial compounds, cloves stand as a fragrant and flavorful addition to the world of herbal remedies, promoting digestion and enhancing overall wellness.

TURMERIC

Turmeric (Curcuma longa) isn't just a vibrant spice; it's a prized herbal remedy celebrated for its radiant color and an impressive array of health benefits. In the realm of digestive health, turmeric shines as a potent ally, offering relief from discomforts and supporting overall well-being.

How Turmeric Supports Digestion:

Turmeric owes its digestive benefits to its star compound, curcumin. Curcumin possesses anti-inflammatory, antioxidant, and antimicrobial properties that work in harmony to soothe and nurture the digestive system.

Benefits for Digestive Health

Anti-Inflammatory Relief: Turmeric's curcumin can help reduce inflammation in the digestive tract, making it beneficial for conditions like irritable bowel syndrome (IBS) and inflammatory bowel disease (IBD).

Aid for Indigestion: Turmeric can stimulate bile production, aiding in the digestion of fats and alleviating symptoms of indigestion such as bloating and discomfort.

Soothing for Gas and Bloating: Turmeric's anti-inflammatory properties can help ease gas and bloating by calming the digestive tract.

Support for Gut Health: Turmeric's antimicrobial properties can help maintain a healthy balance of gut microorganisms, supporting overall gut health.

Ways to Enjoy Turmeric

Golden Milk: A soothing beverage made with turmeric, milk (dairy or plant-based), and spices like black pepper and cinnamon.

Turmeric in Cooking: Incorporate turmeric into your cooking, adding it to curries, rice dishes, soups, and more.

Turmeric Supplements: Curcumin supplements are available, but consuming turmeric in its natural form is often more beneficial due to the presence of other compounds that enhance absorption.

Precautions

While turmeric is generally safe, consuming excessive amounts can lead to stomach upset or interact with certain medications. If you're pregnant, nursing, have gallbladder issues, or are on blood-thinning medications, consult a healthcare professional before using turmeric in medicinal amounts or taking supplements.

Turmeric's radiant hue and exceptional properties make it a shining star in the realm of herbal remedies. With its array of beneficial effects on digestion and overall health, turmeric stands as a golden elixir for promoting digestive harmony and nurturing well-being.

GARLIC

Garlic (Allium sativum) isn't just a pungent spice; it's a revered herbal remedy celebrated for its unique flavor and a myriad of health benefits. In the realm of digestive health, garlic stands as a powerful ally, offering relief from discomforts and supporting overall digestive well-being.

How Garlic Benefits Digestion

Garlic's potent properties come from its bioactive compounds, particularly allicin. Allicin contributes to garlic's antimicrobial, anti-inflammatory, and antioxidant effects, making it a dynamic choice for promoting digestive health.

Benefits for Digestive Health

Support for Gut Microbiota: Garlic's antimicrobial properties can help maintain a balanced gut microbiota, supporting overall gut health.

Aid for Indigestion: Garlic's compounds can stimulate digestive enzymes, aiding in the digestion of foods and alleviating symptoms of indigestion.

Soothing for Bloating and Gas: Garlic's natural carminative properties can help reduce bloating, gas, and abdominal discomfort.

Anti-Inflammatory Relief: Garlic's anti-inflammatory effects can offer relief for conditions like irritable bowel syndrome (IBS) by reducing inflammation in the digestive tract.

Ways to Incorporate Garlic

Cooking with Garlic: Adding fresh or cooked garlic to your meals can infuse dishes with its unique flavor and therapeutic benefits.

Garlic Supplements: Aged garlic supplements, rich in antioxidants, offer benefits without the pungent odor. Consult a healthcare professional before using supplements.

Precautions

Garlic is generally safe, but consuming excessive amounts might lead to stomach upset. If you're pregnant, nursing, have blood-clotting disorders, or are on blood-thinning medications, consult a healthcare professional before using garlic in medicinal amounts or taking supplements.

Garlic's bold presence and multifaceted benefits make it an invaluable addition to the realm of herbal remedies. With its remarkable array of properties for promoting digestion and overall well-being, garlic remains a flavorful and timeless choice for digestive harmony.

ROSEMARY

Rosemary (Rosmarinus officinalis) isn't just a fragrant herb; it's a treasured botanical known for its aromatic allure and an array of health benefits. In the realm of digestive health, rosemary stands as an intriguing ally, offering relief from discomforts and supporting overall well-being.

How Rosemary Nurtures Digestion

Rosemary's benefits come from its bioactive compounds, including rosmarinic acid and essential oils. These compounds contribute to its antioxidant, anti-inflammatory, and carminative effects, making rosemary a dynamic choice for promoting digestive comfort.

Benefits for Digestive Health

Aid for Indigestion: Rosemary's carminative properties can help alleviate symptoms of indigestion, including bloating and discomfort.

Anti-Inflammatory Relief: Rosemary's anti-inflammatory effects can offer support for conditions like irritable bowel syndrome (IBS) by reducing inflammation in the digestive tract.

Calming Effect: The aroma of rosemary can have a calming effect on the stomach, offering relief from nausea and indigestion.

Ways to Embrace Rosemary

Cooking with Rosemary: Adding fresh or dried rosemary to your culinary creations can infuse dishes with its aromatic flavor and therapeutic benefits.

Rosemary Tea: Infusing rosemary leaves in hot water to create a fragrant tea can offer comfort and promote digestion.

Aromatherapy: Inhaling the scent of rosemary essential oil can have a soothing effect on the digestive system.

Precautions

Rosemary is generally safe, but consuming excessive amounts might lead to stomach upset. If you're pregnant, nursing, have epilepsy, or are on medications, consult a healthcare professional before using rosemary in medicinal amounts or in the form of essential oil.

Rosemary's aromatic charm and potential benefits make it a captivating addition to the world of herbal remedies. With its unique blend of properties for promoting digestion and overall well-being, rosemary offers an aromatic embrace to the digestive journey.

OREGANO

Oregano (Origanum vulgare) isn't just a kitchen staple; it's a versatile herb celebrated for its robust flavor and an impressive range of health benefits. In the realm of digestive health, oregano stands as a flavorful ally, offering relief from discomforts and supporting overall well-being.

How Oregano Supports Digestion

Oregano's benefits stem from its bioactive compounds, including carvacrol and thymol. These compounds contribute to oregano's antimicrobial, anti-inflammatory, and antioxidant effects, making it a valuable choice for promoting digestive comfort.

Benefits for Digestive Health

Support for Gut Health: Oregano's antimicrobial properties can help maintain a balanced gut microbiota, supporting overall digestive wellness.

Aid for Indigestion: Oregano's carminative properties can help alleviate symptoms of indigestion, including bloating and discomfort.

Anti-Inflammatory Relief: Oregano's anti-inflammatory effects can provide support for conditions like irritable bowel syndrome (IBS) by reducing inflammation in the digestive tract.

Ways to Enjoy Oregano

Cooking with Oregano: Adding fresh or dried oregano to your culinary creations, from pasta sauces to roasted vegetables, can infuse dishes with its aromatic flavor and therapeutic benefits.

Oregano Oil: Oregano essential oil, when used with caution and under the guidance of a healthcare professional, can offer concentrated benefits.

Precautions

Oregano is generally safe when used in culinary amounts, but consuming excessive amounts of oregano oil might lead to stomach upset. If you're pregnant, nursing, have allergies to plants in the Lamiaceae family (mint family), or are on medications, consult a healthcare professional before using oregano oil or supplements.

Oregano's bold flavor and multifaceted benefits make it an essential addition to the world of herbal remedies. With its remarkable array of properties for promoting digestion and overall well-being, oregano remains a flavorful and versatile choice for digestive harmony.

CHAPTER 3

HOME REMEDIES AND DIY PRACTICES

Homemade Digestive Herbal Teas

Discover the soothing embrace of homemade digestive herbal teas, each crafted with care and blended from nature's bounty. These teas harness the power of various herbs to provide relief from discomforts and promote digestive harmony. Sip and savor the flavors of well-being with these recipes.

Indulge in the therapeutic world of homemade digestive herbal teas, each uniquely crafted to provide comfort, alleviate discomfort, and nurture your digestive well-being. As you brew these delightful blends, savor the soothing qualities of nature's gift and sip your way to wellness.

Peppermint Soothe Tea:

Ingredients:

- 1 teaspoon dried peppermint leaves

- 1 cup hot water

Instructions:

1. Place the dried peppermint leaves in a teapot or cup.

2. Pour hot water over the leaves.

3. Cover and steep for about 5-10 minutes.

4. Strain and enjoy the refreshing and soothing aroma of peppermint.

Chamomile Comfort Tea:

Ingredients:

- 1 teaspoon dried chamomile flowers

- 1 cup hot water

Instructions:

1. Place the dried chamomile flowers in a teapot or cup.

2. Pour hot water over the flowers.

3. Cover and steep for about 5-10 minutes.

4. Strain and relish the gentle and calming effects of chamomile.

Fennel Fusion Tea

Ingredients:

- 1 teaspoon fennel seeds

- 1 teaspoon dried chamomile flowers

- 1 cup hot water

Instructions:

1. Crush the fennel seeds slightly to release their flavors.

2. Place the fennel seeds and dried chamomile flowers in a teapot or cup.

3. Pour hot water over the mixture.

4. Cover and steep for about 5-10 minutes.

5. Strain and experience the fusion of fennel's carminative properties with chamomile's calming touch.

Ginger Elixir Tea:

Ingredients:

- 1 teaspoon grated fresh ginger

- 1 teaspoon dried lemon balm leaves

- 1 cup hot water

Instructions:

1. Place the grated fresh ginger and dried lemon balm leaves in a teapot or cup.

2. Pour hot water over the mixture.

3. Cover and steep for about 5-10 minutes.

4. Strain and enjoy the zesty warmth of ginger combined with the soothing qualities of lemon balm.

Turmeric Wellness Tea

Ingredients:

- 1 teaspoon ground turmeric

- ½ teaspoon ground cinnamon

- Pinch of black pepper

- 1 cup hot water

- Honey (optional)

Instructions:

1. Combine the ground turmeric, ground cinnamon, and a pinch of black pepper in a teapot or cup.

2. Pour hot water over the mixture.

3. Cover and steep for about 5 minutes.

4. Strain and add honey if desired, savoring the golden elixir of turmeric's anti-inflammatory properties.

Rosemary Revive Tea:

Ingredients:

- 1 teaspoon dried rosemary leaves

- 1 teaspoon dried lemon verbena leaves

- 1 cup hot water

Instructions:

1. Place the dried rosemary leaves and dried lemon verbena leaves in a teapot or cup.

2. Pour hot water over the mixture.

3. Cover and steep for about 5-10 minutes.

4. Strain and relish the aromatic harmony of rosemary and lemon verbena.

Oregano Infusion Tea:

Ingredients:

- 1 teaspoon dried oregano leaves

- 1 teaspoon dried thyme leaves

- 1 cup hot water

Instructions:

1. Place the dried oregano leaves and dried thyme leaves in a teapot or cup.

2. Pour hot water over the mixture.

3. Cover and steep for about 5-10 minutes.

4. Strain and savor the robust blend of oregano and thyme.

Infused Water Recipes

Infused water can be a delightful and healthful way to support your digestive system. The following infused water recipes incorporate ingredients known for their digestive benefits, helping to ease discomfort and promote overall well-being. These infusions not only taste great but also provide a gentle boost to your digestive health:

1. **Lemon and Ginger Digestive Elixir**

Ingredients:

- Slices of fresh lemon

- Thinly sliced fresh ginger

- Cold water

Instructions:

1. Fill a pitcher with cold water.

2. Add slices of fresh lemon and thinly sliced ginger.

3. Allow the flavors to infuse for at least an hour, preferably overnight in the refrigerator.

4. Serve chilled for a zesty and soothing digestive elixir.

2. **Minty Cucumber Cool Down**:

Ingredients:

- Fresh mint leaves

- Slices of cucumber

- Cold water

Instructions:

1. Fill a pitcher with cold water.

2. Add fresh mint leaves and slices of cucumber.

3. Allow the flavors to infuse for at least an hour.

4. Serve cold for a refreshing and digestive-friendly treat.

3. **Fennel and Orange Digestive Refresher**

Ingredients:

- Slices of fresh orange

- Crushed fennel seeds (use a mortar and pestle)

- Cold water

Instructions:

1. Fill a pitcher with cold water.

2. Add slices of fresh orange and crushed fennel seeds.

3. Allow the flavors to infuse for at least an hour.

4. Serve cold for a tangy and digestive-refreshing infusion.

4. **Cinnamon Apple Comfort Water**

Ingredients:

- Slices of fresh apple (with the skin)

- A cinnamon stick

- Cold water

Instructions:

1. Fill a pitcher with cold water.

2. Add slices of fresh apple and a cinnamon stick.

3. Allow the flavors to infuse for at least an hour.

4. Serve chilled for a comforting and digestive-friendly beverage.

5. **Papaya and Basil Digestive Bliss**

Ingredients:

- Cubes of fresh papaya

- Fresh basil leaves

- Cold water

Instructions:

1. Fill a pitcher with cold water.

2. Add cubes of fresh papaya and fresh basil leaves.

3. Allow the flavors to infuse for at least an hour.

4. Serve cold for a tropical and digestive-blissful infusion.

6. **Rosemary and Blueberry Digestive Infusion**

Ingredients:

- Fresh rosemary sprigs

- Fresh blueberries

- Cold water

Instructions:

1. Fill a pitcher with cold water.

2. Add fresh rosemary sprigs and fresh blueberries.

3. Allow the flavors to infuse for at least an hour.

4. Serve chilled for a vibrant and digestive-infused treat.

These infused water recipes are not only tasty but also incorporate ingredients known for their digestive-boosting properties. Lemon, ginger, mint, fennel, and other natural elements work harmoniously to support your digestive health. Experiment with these recipes and customize them to your taste preferences for a refreshing and digestive-friendly hydration experience.

Essential Oils for Digestion

Essential oils are potent extracts from aromatic plants that can be used to ease digestive discomfort, promote healthy digestion, and provide overall digestive support. Here are some DIY essential oil blends to help you find natural relief for common digestive issues.

Digestive Soothe Blend:

Ingredients:

- 3 drops Peppermint essential oil

- 2 drops Ginger essential oil

- 2 drops Fennel essential oil

- 1 tablespoon carrier oil (e.g., fractionated coconut oil)

Instructions:

1. In a small glass bottle, combine the essential oils with the carrier oil.

2. Mix well.

3. Massage a few drops of the blend onto your abdomen in a clockwise direction to promote healthy digestion.

Calming Chamomile Blend

Ingredients:

- 3 drops Roman Chamomile essential oil

- 2 drops Lavender essential oil

- 2 drops Lemon essential oil

- 1 tablespoon carrier oil

Instructions:

1. In a small glass bottle, combine the essential oils with the carrier oil.

2. Mix well.

3. Rub a few drops of the blend onto your abdomen to soothe digestive discomfort.

Anti-Bloating Citrus Blend

Ingredients:

- 3 drops Peppermint essential oil

- 2 drops Lemon essential oil

- 2 drops Cardamom essential oil

- 1 tablespoon carrier oil

Instructions:

1. In a small glass bottle, combine the essential oils with the carrier oil.

2. Mix well.

3. Apply a few drops of the blend to your abdomen to alleviate bloating and gas.

Nausea Relief Blend:

Ingredients:

- 3 drops Ginger essential oil

- 2 drops Spearmint essential oil

- 2 drops Lemon essential oil

- 1 tablespoon carrier oil

Instructions:

1. In a small glass bottle, combine the essential oils with the carrier oil.

2. Mix well.

3. Inhale the aroma of the blend from the bottle or apply a drop or two to your wrists and inhale deeply to ease nausea.

Stomach Comfort Blend

Ingredients:

- 3 drops Cardamom essential oil

- 2 drops Peppermint essential oil

- 2 drops Roman Chamomile essential oil

- 1 tablespoon carrier oil

Instructions:

1. In a small glass bottle, combine the essential oils with the carrier oil.

2. Mix well.

3. Gently massage the blend onto your abdomen to relieve stomach discomfort.

DIY Digestive Aid Inhaler:

Ingredients:

- A small inhaler tube with a wick

- 3 drops Peppermint essential oil

- 2 drops Ginger essential oil

- 2 drops Lemon essential oil

Instructions:

1. Place the drops of essential oil onto the wick inside the inhaler tube.

2. Assemble the inhaler and close it tightly.

3. Inhale deeply through each nostril as needed to alleviate digestive discomfort or nausea.

Essential oils are highly concentrated and should be used with caution. Always dilute them with a carrier oil before applying to the skin. If you're pregnant, nursing, have underlying health conditions, or take medications, consult a qualified aromatherapist or healthcare professional before using essential oils for digestion.

These DIY essential oil blends offer natural relief and support for various digestive issues. Whether you prefer massage oils or inhalers, these recipes provide you with options to soothe discomfort and promote healthy digestion using the power of aromatherapy.

CHAPTER 4

DIETARY CHANGES FOR BETTER DIGESTION

Digestion is a complex and intricate process that plays a vital role in our overall well-being. The foods we consume are not only a source of nourishment but also the foundation of a healthy digestive system. Making mindful dietary changes can significantly impact how our bodies process and absorb nutrients, leading to better digestion and improved quality of life.

In this exploration of dietary changes for better digestion, we embark on a journey to discover the power of nutrition in maintaining digestive health. From choosing the right foods to adopting smarter eating habits, this guide will provide valuable insights into transforming your relationship with food.

We will delve into the world of dietary fiber, explore the benefits of hydration, and uncover the wonders of probiotics.

As we navigate this dietary landscape, we'll empower ourselves with knowledge and practical strategies to nurture our digestive systems. By the end, you'll be equipped with the tools needed to make dietary choices that promote better digestion, enhance nutrient absorption, and foster a harmonious connection between body and food.

DIETARY FIBER

Dietary fiber is a powerhouse nutrient that significantly contributes to better digestion and overall health. It's the part of plant-based foods that your body can't digest or absorb, but it plays a crucial role in maintaining a healthy digestive system.

Digestive Benefits of Dietary Fiber

Regulating Bowel Movements: Fiber adds bulk to your stool, making it easier to pass, which helps prevent constipation. It can also aid in managing diarrhea by absorbing excess water.

Promoting Gut Health: Certain types of fiber, known as prebiotics, act as food for beneficial gut bacteria. This helps maintain a balanced gut microbiome, which is essential for digestion and overall well-being. ***Preventing Hemorrhoids and Diverticulosis***: Fiber's ability to keep stools soft and easy to pass reduces the risk of hemorrhoids and diverticulosis, conditions related to straining during bowel movements.

Lowering the Risk of Colon Cancer: High-fiber diets have been linked to a reduced risk of colorectal cancer, possibly due to fiber's role in keeping the digestive tract healthy and promoting regular bowel movements.

Sources of Dietary Fiber

Whole Grains: Foods like brown rice, whole wheat bread, and oats are rich in fiber. Opt for whole grains over

refined grains for better digestive
health.

Legumes: Beans, lentils, and chickpeas
are excellent sources of fiber and
plant-based protein.

Fruits and Vegetables: Apples, pears,
broccoli, carrots, and leafy greens are
fiber-packed choices.

Nuts and Seeds: Almonds, chia seeds,
and flaxseeds are fiber-rich additions
to your diet.

Tips for Increasing Dietary Fiber

- Increase your fiber intake
  gradually to allow your digestive
  system to adjust.
- Fiber absorbs water, so it's
  essential to drink enough fluids
  to keep your stools soft.
- Diverse Diet: Consume a variety
  of fiber sources to benefit from

different types of fiber and nutrients.

- Read Labels: When shopping for packaged foods, check the nutrition labels for the fiber content.

Dietary fiber is a key player in maintaining digestive health. By incorporating fiber-rich foods into your diet and staying mindful of your overall nutrition, you can promote better digestion, prevent digestive issues, and support your long-term well-being.

PROBIOTIC-RICH FOOD

Probiotics are living microorganisms, often referred to as "good" or "friendly" bacteria, that offer numerous benefits for your digestive system. Consuming probiotic-rich foods can enhance the balance of these beneficial microbes in your gut and promote better digestion and overall well-being.

Digestive Benefits of Probiotic-Rich Foods

Improved Gut Health: Probiotics contribute to a healthy gut microbiome by increasing the abundance of beneficial bacteria. A balanced gut microbiome is essential for efficient digestion.

Enhanced Nutrient Absorption: Probiotics help your body absorb nutrients more effectively, ensuring you get the most out of the foods you eat.

Reduced Digestive Discomfort: Probiotics can alleviate symptoms of irritable bowel syndrome (IBS), including bloating, gas, and abdominal discomfort.

Protection Against Diarrhea: Probiotics are known to be effective in preventing and treating diarrhea, particularly when caused by infections or antibiotic use.

Constipation Relief: Certain probiotic strains can help regulate bowel movements and ease constipation.

Probiotic-Rich Foods to Incorporate

Yogurt: Contains live and active cultures of beneficial bacteria. Look for yogurt with "live and active cultures" on the label.

Kefir: A fermented milk drink rich in probiotics. It's similar to yogurt but has a thinner consistency.

Sauerkraut: Fermented cabbage that's a good source of probiotics. Ensure it's raw and unpasteurized for live cultures.

Kimchi: A spicy Korean dish made from fermented vegetables, typically cabbage and radishes.

Miso: A traditional Japanese seasoning made from fermented soybeans or grains, often used in soups.

Tempeh: A fermented soybean product with a nutty flavor and firm texture, often used in vegetarian and vegan dishes.

Pickles: Naturally fermented pickles (not vinegar-pickled) can contain probiotics.

Tips for Incorporating Probiotics

- Consume a variety of probiotic-rich foods to introduce different strains of beneficial bacteria into your gut.
- Check product labels to ensure they contain live cultures, and avoid overly processed versions that may have lost their probiotic content.

- While probiotics are beneficial,
  don't overconsume them. A
  balanced diet with a mix of fiber
  and nutrients is crucial for gut
  health.
- Combine with Prebiotics foods,
  like garlic, onions, and bananas,
  feed the probiotics, enhancing
  their effectiveness.

By incorporating probiotic-rich foods
into your diet, you can nurture a
healthy gut microbiome, which, in
turn, supports better digestion,
nutrient absorption, and overall
digestive wellness.

HYDRATION AND DIGESTION

The relationship between hydration and digestion is profound and pivotal for overall well-being. Water is not only essential for life but also plays a critical role in every step of the digestive process. Understanding this connection can help you maintain a healthy digestive system.

How Hydration Impacts Digestion:

Saliva Production: The digestive process begins in the mouth, where enzymes in saliva help break down food. Proper hydration ensures an adequate flow of saliva, facilitating the initial stages of digestion.

Enzyme Activation: Digestive enzymes in the stomach and small intestine rely on water to function effectively.

Adequate hydration helps these enzymes break down food into smaller particles for absorption.

Nutrient Absorption: Water aids in the absorption of nutrients in the small intestine. It helps transport these nutrients into the bloodstream, making them available for your body's needs.

Prevention of Constipation: Dehydration can lead to hard, dry stools, contributing to constipation. Sufficient water intake keeps stools soft and easy to pass, preventing constipation.

Reduced Risk of Acid Reflux: Proper hydration helps maintain the mucosal lining of the esophagus, reducing the risk of acid reflux and heartburn.

How Much Water Is Needed:

The recommended daily water intake varies but generally falls within 8 to 10 cups (64 to 80 ounces) for most adults. However, individual needs can differ based on factors like age, activity level, and climate.

Tips for Staying Hydrated:

- **Regular Sips**: Sip water throughout the day rather than relying on infrequent large glasses.
- **Monitor Urine Color**: Aim for pale yellow urine, a sign of adequate hydration. Dark yellow or amber urine may indicate dehydration.

- **Hydrate with Meals**: Drink water before, during, and after meals to aid digestion.
- **Incorporate Hydrating Foods**: Foods like watermelon, cucumbers, and oranges have high water content and contribute to hydration.
- **Listen to Your Body**: Thirst is a natural indicator of dehydration. Pay attention to your body's cues and respond accordingly.

- **Consider Electrolytes:** In cases of heavy sweating (e.g., exercise or hot weather), replenish electrolytes lost through drinks like sports beverages.

Proper hydration is integral to maintaining a well-functioning digestive system. By drinking enough water and being mindful of your body's needs, you can promote efficient digestion, prevent discomfort, and support your overall health.

CHAPTER 5

LIFESTYLE TIPS

Digestive health is the cornerstone of our well-being, and its balance is influenced not only by the foods we eat but also by the way we live. Lifestyle choices play a significant role in how our digestive system functions. This guide explores a range of practical and holistic lifestyle tips to help you nurture and maintain a harmonious digestive system.

From stress management techniques that ease the burden on your gut to physical activity that keeps your digestive tract active and healthy, we delve into the multifaceted aspects of daily life that impact how we digest, absorb nutrients, and eliminate waste.

We'll explore the importance of mindful eating, emphasizing the quality of your meals over quantity. We'll discuss the significance of adequate sleep in supporting optimal digestive function and explore how staying active is essential not just for overall health but for the digestive process itself.

By the end of this journey, you'll be armed with a wealth of knowledge and practical strategies to integrate into your daily life. These lifestyle tips aren't just about nurturing your digestive health; they're about embracing a holistic approach to well-being, where mind, body, and digestive system work in harmony to promote your overall health and vitality.

MINDFUL EATING

Mindful eating is a practice that encourages full awareness and presence during meals. It involves paying close attention to the sensory aspects of eating, recognizing hunger and fullness cues, and fostering a non-judgmental attitude toward food. Mindful eating is a holistic approach that benefits not only your mental well-being but also your digestive health.

Benefits of Mindful Eating for Digestive Health

Improved Digestion: Mindful eating promotes slower, more deliberate chewing, which assists the digestive process. When you chew food thoroughly, your stomach has an easier time breaking it down.

Enhanced Nutrient Absorption: By savoring each bite and focusing on your meal, you increase the absorption of essential nutrients from your food.
Reduced Overeating: Mindful eating helps you recognize when you're truly hungry and when you're comfortably full, reducing the likelihood of overeating or undereating.

Better Food Choices: Increased awareness of your body's needs and cravings allows you to make more mindful and nutritious food choices.
Less Digestive Discomfort: Eating mindfully can reduce symptoms of indigestion, bloating, and heartburn by preventing the consumption of food when stressed or distracted.

How to Practice Mindful Eating:

- Engage Your Senses:

 Observe the colors, smells, and textures of your food. Take time to appreciate the aesthetics of your meal.

- Chew Thoroughly:

Aim to chew each bite at least 20-30 times. This enhances digestion and allows you to fully taste your food.

- Eliminate Distractions:

Turn off the TV, put away electronic devices, and create a peaceful eating environment. Avoid eating in a rush.

- Pause and Reflect:

Take breaks between bites. Put down your utensils, and breathe deeply.

Assess your level of hunger and fullness.

- Listen to Your Body:

Pay attention to hunger and fullness cues. Eat when you're hungry, and stop when you're satisfied.

- Eat Consciously:

Enjoy the experience of eating without judgment. Be aware of any emotional triggers that may influence your eating habits.

- Appreciate Your Food:

Express gratitude for the nourishment your meal provides. Cultivate a positive attitude toward food.

- Start Small:

Begin by incorporating mindful eating into one meal per day. Gradually expand this practice to all your meals.

- Practice Mindful Snacking:

Extend mindful eating to snacks as well. Opt for nutritious, satisfying choices that align with your hunger cues.

- Seek Support: Consider joining a mindfulness or mindful eating group or consulting with a registered dietitian who specializes in mindful eating.

Mindful eating is a lifelong journey that can enhance your digestive health, foster a positive relationship with food, and contribute to overall well-being. By savoring each meal and paying attention to your body's signals, you can make more conscious food choices and create a sense of balance in your eating habits.

EXERCISE

Digestive health isn't solely influenced by what you eat; it's also profoundly impacted by your physical activity levels. Exercise offers a multitude of benefits that positively affect your digestive system and overall well-being. Here's a comprehensive look at why exercise is crucial for digestive health

Enhanced Bowel Regularity:

Exercise helps stimulate the muscles of the digestive tract, promoting the movement of food and waste through your system. This can alleviate or prevent constipation.

Reduced Risk of Digestive Disorders:

Engaging in regular physical activity is associated with a decreased risk of digestive issues such as diverticulitis, gallstones, and colorectal cancer.

Weight Management:

Maintaining a healthy weight through exercise can prevent or alleviate obesity-related digestive conditions like acid reflux and fatty liver disease.

Stress Reduction

Stress can negatively impact digestive health. Exercise is a powerful stress reducer, which can help manage conditions like irritable bowel syndrome (IBS).

Improved Gut Microbiome:

Physical activity is linked to a more diverse and balanced gut microbiome.

A healthy gut microbiome is vital for optimal digestion and overall health.

Better Blood Sugar Control:

Exercise helps regulate blood sugar levels, reducing the risk of type 2 diabetes, which can have adverse effects on digestion.

Enhanced Nutrient Absorption:

 Regular exercise increases blood flow to the digestive tract, improving the absorption of essential nutrients from your food.

Reduction of Gas and Bloating:

Exercise can alleviate symptoms of gas and bloating by aiding the movement of gas through the digestive system.

Prevention of Colon Cancer:

Regular physical activity has been linked to a lower risk of colon cancer, possibly due to its beneficial effects on bowel regularity and inflammation.

How to Incorporate Exercise for Digestive Health

- Cardiovascular Exercise: Activities like walking, jogging, cycling, and swimming can get your heart rate up and promote overall digestive health.
- Strength Training: Building muscle through weightlifting or bodyweight exercises can enhance metabolic function, which supports digestion.
- Yoga: This practice combines physical movement with relaxation techniques, reducing stress and promoting gut health.
- Stretching: Gentle stretching exercises like yoga or Pilates can

ease tension in the abdominal region, aiding digestion.

- Consistency: Aim for at least 150 minutes of moderate-intensity aerobic activity or 75 minutes of vigorous-intensity aerobic activity per week, along with muscle-strengthening activities on two or more days per week.

Remember to consult with a healthcare professional or fitness expert before starting a new exercise regimen, especially if you have underlying health conditions. By incorporating regular exercise into your routine, you can support your digestive health, reduce the risk of digestive disorders, and enjoy a more vibrant and balanced life.

YOGA

Yoga is a holistic practice that benefits not only your physical and mental well-being but also plays a significant role in promoting digestive health. By incorporating yoga into your routine, you can enhance digestion, alleviate common digestive issues, and foster overall gut health. Here's a comprehensive guide to yoga for digestive well-being:

How Yoga Supports Digestive Health

Stress Reduction: Yoga encourages relaxation and reduces stress, which is vital for digestive health. High stress levels can lead to digestive discomfort and conditions like irritable bowel syndrome (IBS).

Improved Blood Flow: Yoga poses and deep breathing techniques enhance blood circulation, including to the digestive organs. This supports optimal digestion and nutrient absorption.

Stimulates Digestive Organs: Specific yoga poses target the abdominal area, such as twists and forward bends, which massage and stimulate the digestive organs, aiding in digestion.

Enhanced Peristalsis: Yoga poses that involve stretching and contracting the abdominal muscles can improve peristalsis, the rhythmic contraction of the intestines that moves food through the digestive tract.

Yoga Poses for Digestive Health

- Child's Pose (Balasana): This gentle forward bend relaxes the abdominal muscles and can relieve gas and bloating.
- Cat-Cow Pose (Marjaryasana-Bitilasana): The spinal flexion and extension in this pose massages the digestive organs and promotes flexibility in the spine.
- Seated Forward Bend (Paschimottanasana): This pose stretches the entire back of the body, including the digestive organs, promoting peristalsis.
- Twisting Poses (e.g., Bharadvajasana): Twists wring out the abdominal area, massaging and stimulating the digestive organs.

- Downward Dog (Adho Mukha Svanasana): This inversion encourages blood flow to the head and upper body, supporting digestion and reducing stress.
- Wind-Relieving Pose (Pavanamuktasana): This posture compresses the abdomen, aiding in the elimination of gas.

Yoga and Breathwork (Pranayama) for Digestive Health

1. Deep Belly Breathing: Practice deep diaphragmatic breathing to massage and stimulate the digestive organs.

2. Kapalbhati Pranayama: This rapid breathwork technique can

improve digestion by stimulating the abdominal area.
3. Nadi Shodhana (Alternate Nostril Breathing): Balancing the breath through alternate nostrils can reduce stress and promote digestive harmony.

Incorporating Yoga into Your Routine:

- Start with a gentle yoga practice if you're new to yoga or have digestive issues.

- Aim for consistency. Even a few minutes of daily practice can yield benefits.

- Listen to your body. Avoid poses that cause discomfort, and consider props or modifications for support.

- Seek guidance from a certified yoga instructor, especially if you have specific digestive concerns.

Yoga offers a holistic approach to digestive health by addressing both physical and mental aspects. By embracing yoga as part of your lifestyle, you can foster a more balanced and harmonious digestive system, promoting overall well-being.

STRESS MANAGEMENT

The link between stress and digestive health is profound. Chronic stress can wreak havoc on your digestive system, leading to a range of issues like irritable bowel syndrome (IBS), indigestion, and even exacerbating conditions like inflammatory bowel disease. Here's a comprehensive guide on how to manage stress for better digestive health:

Understanding the Stress-Digestion Connection

Stress Hormones: When you're stressed, your body releases stress hormones like cortisol. These hormones can disrupt the normal functioning of your digestive system, slowing down digestion and increasing inflammation.

Alteration of Gut Microbiome: Chronic stress can change the composition of your gut microbiome, affecting digestion and potentially leading to gastrointestinal problems.

Muscle Tension: Stress can cause tension in the muscles of the digestive tract, leading to conditions like cramps, bloating, and constipation.

Effective Stress Management Techniques

1. Mindfulness Meditation: Mindfulness techniques, such as meditation and deep breathing exercises, can reduce stress levels and promote relaxation. Regular practice can help prevent stress-related digestive issues.

2. Regular Exercise: Physical activity is a powerful stress reducer. Engage in regular exercise to release endorphins and ease stress.

3. Yoga: Yoga combines physical postures with mindfulness, making it an excellent stress management tool that also benefits digestion.

4. Balanced Diet: A well-balanced diet can help stabilize blood sugar levels and support mood regulation, reducing the impact of stress on digestion.

5. Adequate Sleep: Prioritize quality sleep to restore your body and reduce stress. Poor sleep can exacerbate digestive problems.

6. Social Support: Lean on friends and family for emotional support. Talking about your stressors can alleviate their impact.

7. Time Management: Efficiently manage your time to reduce stress

from overwhelming workloads and deadlines.

8. Hobbies and Relaxation: Engage in activities you enjoy, whether it's reading, gardening, or listening to music. These hobbies can provide an escape from stress.

9. Professional Help: If stress becomes overwhelming or chronic, consider seeking therapy or counseling to address underlying issues and develop coping strategies.

Stress management is not just beneficial for your mental health; it's vital for your digestive well-being. By implementing these stress-reduction strategies, you can mitigate the harmful effects of stress on your digestive system, promote better digestion, and enjoy improved overall health and vitality.

HEALTHY SLEEP

Quality sleep is essential for overall well-being, and its impact on digestive health is profound. Poor sleep patterns can disrupt the delicate balance of your digestive system, leading to a range of issues like indigestion, acid reflux, and even irritable bowel syndrome (IBS). Here's a comprehensive guide on how to prioritize healthy sleep for better digestive health:

Understanding the Sleep-Digestion Connection

Gut-Brain Axis: The gut and brain are closely connected through the gut-brain axis. Sleep disturbances can disrupt this communication, affecting digestion.

Hormonal Balance: Sleep regulates the release of hormones that influence appetite and metabolism. Poor sleep can lead to imbalances that affect digestion and increase the risk of weight gain.

Inflammation: Chronic sleep deprivation can increase inflammation in the body, which can harm the digestive tract and lead to conditions like inflammatory bowel disease (IBD).

Effective Strategies for Healthy Sleep

- Consistent Sleep Schedule: Go to bed and wake up at the same time every day, even on weekends. Consistency reinforces your body's natural sleep-wake cycle.
- Create a Relaxing Bedtime Routine: Engage in calming activities before bed, such as reading, gentle stretching, or taking a warm bath, to signal to your body that it's time to wind down.
- Sleep-Inducing Environment: Make your sleep environment comfortable and conducive to rest. A cool, dark, and quiet room is ideal.

- Limit Screen Time: Avoid screens (phones, tablets, computers, and TVs) at least an hour before bedtime. The blue light emitted can interfere with melatonin production, a hormone crucial for sleep.
- Mindfulness and Relaxation Techniques: Practices like meditation, deep breathing exercises, or progressive muscle relaxation can help calm your mind and prepare it for sleep.
- Limit Caffeine and Alcohol: Avoid caffeine and alcohol close to bedtime, as they can disrupt sleep patterns.
- Regular Exercise: Engaging in regular physical activity can promote better sleep, but avoid vigorous exercise close to bedtime.

- Balanced Diet: Avoid heavy or spicy meals close to bedtime, as they can lead to indigestion and disrupt sleep.

Prioritizing healthy sleep patterns is not just beneficial for your mental and physical well-being; it's vital for digestive health. By incorporating these sleep-improvement strategies, you can promote better digestion, reduce the risk of digestive disorders, and enjoy improved overall health and vitality.

CHAPTER 6

RECIPES

Here are gut-healing recipes designed to support digestive health. Each recipe includes the ingredients with quantities and step-by-step cooking instructions.

Healing Chicken and Rice Soup

Ingredients:

- 1 cup cooked chicken (shredded)

- 1 cup cooked rice

- 4 cups chicken broth

- 1 carrot (diced)

- 1 celery stalk (diced)

- ½ cup spinach (chopped)

- ½ teaspoon turmeric

- Salt and pepper to taste

Instructions:

1. In a large pot, heat the chicken broth over medium heat.

2. Add diced carrot and celery. Simmer for 10 minutes until they soften.

3. Stir in cooked chicken, cooked rice, and turmeric.

4. Simmer for another 5-10 minutes until heated through.

5. Add chopped spinach and season with salt and pepper.

6. Serve hot, soothing your digestive tract.

Gut-Friendly Oatmeal

Ingredients:

- 1 cup rolled oats

- 2 cups water

- 1 banana (sliced)

- 1 tablespoon honey

- ½ teaspoon ground cinnamon

- A handful of sliced almonds

Instructions:

1. Combine oats and water in a saucepan and cook according to package instructions.

2. Once cooked, top with banana slices, honey, cinnamon, and sliced almonds.

3. Enjoy this fiber-rich breakfast to support digestion.

Gut-Healing Smoothie

Ingredients:

- 1 cup Greek yogurt

- ½ cup mixed berries (blueberries, strawberries, raspberries)

- 1 ripe banana

- 1 tablespoon honey

- 1 tablespoon ground flaxseed

- ½ cup spinach

- ½ cup water or almond milk

Instructions:

1. Blend all ingredients until smooth.

2. Adjust liquid as needed to achieve your desired consistency.

3. Sip this nutrient-packed smoothie for a gut-friendly breakfast or snack.

Roasted Sweet Potato and Chickpea Salad

Ingredients:

- 2 sweet potatoes (cubed)

- 1 can chickpeas (drained and rinsed)

- 2 tablespoons olive oil

- 1 teaspoon cumin

- Salt and pepper to taste

- Mixed greens

- Lemon-tahini dressing

Instructions:

1. Toss sweet potato cubes and chickpeas in olive oil, cumin, salt, and pepper.

2. Roast in the oven at 400°F (200°C) for 25-30 minutes.

3. Serve on a bed of mixed greens and drizzle with lemon-tahini dressing.

Ginger and Turmeric Tea

Ingredients:

- 1-inch piece of fresh ginger (sliced)

- 1 teaspoon ground turmeric

- 1 teaspoon honey

- 2 cups hot water

Instructions:

1. Combine ginger, turmeric, and honey in a teapot.

2. Pour hot water over the mixture.

3. Let it steep for 5-10 minutes.

4. Strain and sip on this soothing tea to ease digestive discomfort.

Baked Salmon with Lemon and Dill

Ingredients:

- 4 salmon fillets

- 2 tablespoons olive oil

- Zest and juice of 1 lemon

- 2 cloves garlic (minced)

- 1 tablespoon fresh dill (chopped)

- Salt and pepper to taste

Instructions:

1. Preheat the oven to 375°F (190°C).

2. In a bowl, mix olive oil, lemon zest, lemon juice, garlic, dill, salt, and pepper.

3. Place salmon fillets on a baking sheet, and brush with the lemon-dill mixture.

4. Bake for 15-20 minutes until salmon flakes easily.

5. Serve with steamed vegetables for a nourishing meal.

Quinoa and Vegetable Stir-Fry

Ingredients:

- 1 cup quinoa (cooked)

- 2 tablespoons sesame oil

- 1 bell pepper (sliced)

- 1 cup broccoli florets

- 1 cup snap peas

- 1 carrot (sliced)

- 2 cloves garlic (minced)

- 2 tablespoons low-sodium soy sauce

- 1 tablespoon honey

- 1 teaspoon grated fresh ginger

Instructions

1. Heat sesame oil in a large pan or wok.

2. Add minced garlic and grated ginger. Sauté for 1 minute.

3. Add sliced bell pepper, broccoli, snap peas, and carrot. Stir-fry for 5-7 minutes until tender-crisp.

4. In a small bowl, mix soy sauce and honey.

5. Add cooked quinoa and the soy sauce-honey mixture to the stir-fry. Stir until everything is heated through.

6. Serve this fiber-rich dish for a satisfying and gut-healthy meal.

Papaya and Greek Yogurt Parfait

Ingredients:

- 1 ripe papaya (cubed and seeded)

- 1 cup Greek yogurt

- 2 tablespoons honey

- A handful of granola

Instructions:

1. Layer cubed papaya, Greek yogurt, and honey in a glass.

2. Top with granola for added fiber and crunch.

3. This parfait is a delightful way to support digestive health.

Cucumber and Mint Infused Water

Ingredients:

- 1 cucumber (sliced)

- A handful of fresh mint leaves

- 2 quarts of water

Instructions:

1. Combine cucumber slices and mint leaves in a pitcher.

2. Fill the pitcher with water.

3. Let it infuse for a few hours or overnight.

4. Stay hydrated with this refreshing drink to support digestion.

Miso Soup

Ingredients:

- 4 cups vegetable or chicken broth

- ¼ cup miso paste

- 1 cup tofu (cubed)

- 1 cup seaweed (sliced)

- 2 green onions (sliced)

Instructions:

1. In a pot, heat the broth until hot but not boiling.

2. In a separate bowl, dissolve miso paste in a small amount of hot broth.

3. Add the dissolved miso paste back into the pot.

4. Add tofu, seaweed, and green onions. Simmer for 5-7 minutes.

5. Serve this probiotic-rich soup to support gut health.

These gut-healing recipes are not only delicious but also nourishing for your digestive system. Incorporate them into your diet to promote optimal digestive health and overall well-being.

CONCLUSION

As we reach the end of this insightful journey into the realm of digestive health, we hope you feel empowered with the knowledge and tools to nurture and revitalize your digestive system. Digestive well-being is a cornerstone of overall health, and by taking proactive steps, you can foster a harmonious relationship with your body, food, and lifestyle.

Throughout this book, we've explored the intricacies of the digestive system, the common digestive issues many face, and the incredible benefits of natural remedies, mindful eating, exercise, stress management, and healthy sleep practices. Armed with this wisdom, you are now better equipped to make informed choices that support your digestive health.

Remember, the path to digestive well-being is not about perfection but progress. Small, sustainable changes can yield significant results. Listen to your body, respect its signals, and approach your digestive journey with kindness and patience.

As you embark on this path, keep in mind that digestive health is intimately connected to your overall well-being. A thriving digestive system is not only a source of physical vitality but also a catalyst for mental and emotional balance. It's the foundation upon which you can build a healthier, more vibrant life.

In closing, we encourage you to embrace the power of holistic digestive well-being. Share your newfound knowledge with others, and together, let's cultivate a world where we all prioritize and celebrate the incredible gift of a well-functioning digestive system. May your digestive journey be one of fulfillment, nourishment, and lifelong vitality.

www.ingramcontent.com/pod-product-compliance
Lightning Source LLC
Chambersburg PA
CBHW070941260726
48661CB00003B/1069